How To Easily Improve

Ray Williams

INTRODUCTION

Orlistat obstructs a portion of the fat that you eat, holding it back from being consumed by your body.

Orlistat is utilized to support weight reduction, or to assist with lessening the gamble of recapturing weight previously lost. This medication should be utilized along with a diminished calorie diet and expanded active work. Orlistat is for utilize just in grown-ups that are overweight or corpulent.

Alerts

Try not to take orlistat in the event that you are pregnant.

You shouldn't utilize this medication in the event that you have a stomach related jumble (issues retaining food). You shouldn't utilize Xenical in the event that you have gallbladder issues, or on the other hand assuming you are pregnant. Try not to utilize Alli on the off chance that you have had an organ relocate, assuming you use cyclosporine, or on the other hand in the event that you are not overweight.

Orlistat is just important for a total program of treatment that likewise incorporates diet, exercise, and weight control. Your day to day admission of fat, protein, and carbs ought to be equitably isolated over your everyday feasts as a whole. Follow your eating regimen, prescription, and work-out schedules intently.

Keep away from an eating regimen that is high in fat. High-fat dinners taken in blend with orlistat can expand your gamble of upsetting secondary effects on your stomach or digestion tracts.

Prior to taking this medication

You shouldn't utilize orlistat on the off chance that you are sensitive to it, assuming you have malabsorption condition (a powerlessness to retain food and supplements appropriately), or on the other hand in the event that you are pregnant.

You likewise shouldn't utilize Xenical assuming you have:

gallbladder issues; or

in the event that you are pregnant.

Try not to utilize Alli if:

you are not overweight;

you have had an organ relocate; or

you are taking cyclosporine

To ensure orlistat is alright for you, let your primary care physician know if you have at any point had:

kidney stones;

gallbladder illness;

pancreatitis;

thyroid illness;

liver illness;

kidney illness; or

organ relocate; or

a dietary issue (anorexia or bulimia).

Try not to utilize orlistat assuming that you are pregnant. Weight reduction isn't suggested during pregnancy, regardless of whether you are overweight. Quit taking this medication and tell your primary care physician immediately in the event that you become pregnant.

Taking orlistat can make it harder for your body to assimilate specific nutrients. These nutrients are significant on the off chance that you are nursing a child. Try not to utilize this medication without a specialist's recommendation on the off chance that you are bosom taking care of a child.

Xenical isn't supported for use by anybody more youthful than 12 years of age. Try not to give Alli to anybody under 18 years of age.

How might I take orlistat?

Use orlistat precisely as coordinated on the mark, or as recommended by your primary care physician. Try not to use in bigger or more modest sums or for longer than suggested.

Never share orlistat with someone else, particularly somebody with a background marked by dietary problems.

Peruse all quiet data, medicine guides, and guidance sheets gave to you. Inquire as to whether you have any inquiries.

Orlistat is typically required 3 times each day with every principal dinner that contains some fat (something like 30% of the calories for that feast).

You might take the medication either with your feast or as long as 1 hour subsequent to eating.

In the event that you skirt a feast or you eat a dinner that contains no fat, skirt your portion for that dinner.

The fat substance of your day to day diet ought not be more prominent than 30% of your absolute everyday caloric admission. For instance, assuming that you eat 1200 calories each day, something like 360 of those calories ought to be as fat.

Peruse the name of all food things you devour, really focusing on the quantity of servings per compartment. Your primary care physician, sustenance guide, or dietitian can assist you with fostering a smart dieting plan.

Orlistat is just important for a total program of treatment that likewise incorporates diet and exercise. Your day to day admission of fat, protein, and starches ought to be equitably separated over your day to day feasts in general. Follow your eating regimen, prescription, and work-out schedules intently.

Orlistat can make it harder for your body to retain specific nutrients, and you might have to take a nutrient and mineral enhancement while you are taking this medication. Adhere to your primary care physician's guidelines about the sort of supplement to utilize. Take the enhancement at sleep time, or possibly 2 hours prior or after you take orlistat.

Store at room temperature away from dampness, intensity, and light. Keep the container firmly shut. Discard any unused orlistat after the termination date on the medication name has passed.

What occurs in the event that I miss a portion?

Accept the missed portion when you recollect, however something like 1 hour in the wake of eating a feast. In the event that it has been over an hour since your last feast, skirt the missed portion and take the medication at your next consistently booked time. Try not to take additional medication to make up the missed portion.

What occurs assuming that I glut?

Look for crisis clinical consideration or call the Toxic Substance Help line at 1-800-222-1222.

What to stay away from

Abstain from eating high-fat feasts or you could meaningfully affect your stomach or digestion tracts.

Assuming you additionally take cyclosporine, don't take it in the span of 3 hours prior or 3 hours after you take orlistat.

In the event that you additionally take levothyroxine (like Synthroid), don't take it in no less than 4 hours prior or 4 hours after you take orlistat.

Orlistat aftereffects

Get crisis clinical assistance in the event that you have indications of an unfavorably susceptible response to orlistat: hives; troublesome breathing; enlarging of your face, lips, tongue, or throat.

Quit utilizing orlistat and call your PCP immediately on the off chance that you have:

serious stomach torment;

serious torment in your lower back;

blood in your pee, excruciating or troublesome pee;

indications of kidney issues including almost no peeing; enlarging in your feet or lower legs; feeling drained or winded; or

indications of liver issues including sickness, upper stomach torment, tingling, tired feeling, loss of craving, dull pee, dirt shaded stools, jaundice (yellowing of the skin or eyes).

Normal orlistat incidental effects are brought about by its fat-obstructing activity. These are signs that the medication is working appropriately. These secondary effects are typically transitory and may reduce as you keep utilizing this medication:

slick or greasy stools;

slick spotting in your underpants;

orange or earthy colored shaded oil in your stool;

gas and slick release;

diarrheas, or an earnest need to go to the restroom, powerlessness to control solid discharges;

an expanded number of solid discharges; or

stomach torment, queasiness, rectal agony.

Dosing data

Normal Grown-up Portion for Weight:

120 mg orally three times each day with every fundamental feast containing fat. The portion might be taken during the feast or in something like 1 hour of finishing the dinner.

Common Pediatric Portion for Weight:

12 years or more established:

120 mg orally three times each day with every primary feast containing fat. The portion might be taken during the dinner or in the span of 1 hour of finishing the feast.

What different medications will influence orlistat?

Inquire as to whether it is ok for you to utilize orlistat on the off chance that you are likewise utilizing any of the accompanying medications:

amiodarone;

cyclosporine;

insulin or oral diabetes medication;

HIV or Helps drugs;

seizure medication (particularly assuming your seizures deteriorate while taking this medication);

a nutrient or mineral enhancement that contains beta-carotene or vitamin E; or

a blood more slender - warfarin, Coumadin, Jantoven.

This rundown is incomplete. Different medications might communicate with orlistat, including remedy and over-the-counter meds, nutrients, and natural items. Not all potential associations are recorded in this prescription aide.

Legitimate Use

Take this medication just as coordinated by your primary care physician. Try not to take a greater amount of it, don't take it more regularly, and don't take it for a more drawn out time frame than your PCP requested.

This medication accompanies a patient data embed. Peruse and adhere to the directions in the addition cautiously. Converse with your PCP assuming you have any inquiries.

Orlistat forestalls the ingestion of a portion of the fat you eat. You ought to take it with fluids during the feast or as long as 1 hour subsequent to eating. Assuming you infrequently miss a dinner or eat a feast that contains no fat, you ought to skirt the portion of orlistat.

Since orlistat may diminish how much a few nutrients that your body ingests from food, you should take a multivitamin supplement one time per day. Take the nutrient enhancement somewhere around 2 hours prior or in the wake of taking orlistat. You may likewise take your multivitamin supplement at sleep time.

While utilizing orlistat, you're eating regimen ought to contain something like 30% of calories as fat. More fat in your eating routine will build the symptoms of this medication. Your eating routine ought to be healthfully adjusted, and your day to day admission of fat, sugars, and protein ought to be appropriated north of three principal dinners.

Cautiously adhere to your PCP's directions for a diminished calorie diet plan and customary activity. Chat with your primary care physician prior to beginning any activity program.

Assuming you are utilizing cyclosporine (Gengraf®, Neoral®, Sandimmune®) and levothyroxine (Levothroid®, Synthroid®), don't take them while you take this medication. It is ideal to take cyclosporine no less than 3 hours prior or 3 hours subsequent to taking orlistat. Levothyroxine should be utilized somewhere around 4 hours prior or 4 hours after you take orlistat.

Dosing

The portion of this medication will be different for various patients. Follow your physician's instructions or the bearings on the name. The accompanying data incorporates just the normal portions of this medication. Assuming your portion is unique, don't transform it except if your PCP advises you to do as such.

How much medication that you take relies upon the strength of the medication. Likewise, the quantity of portions you require every day, the time permitted among dosages, and the timeframe you take the medication rely upon the clinical issue for which you are utilizing the medication.

For oral measurement structure (cases):

For treatment of corpulence:

Grown-ups and youngsters — 120 milligrams (mg) three times each day with dinners containing fat.

Kids more youthful than 12 years old — Use and portion not entirely set in stone by your primary care physician.

Missed Portion

In the event that you miss a portion of this medication, skirt the missed portion and return to your standard dosing plan. Don't twofold portions.

Capacity

Store the medication in a shut holder at room temperature, away from intensity, dampness, and direct light. Hold back from freezing.

Keep out of the range of youngsters.

Try not to keep obsolete medication or medication at this point not required.

Ask your medical care proficient how you ought to discard any medication you don't utilize.

Wegovy (semaglutide) infusion is a physician endorsed medication utilized for weight reduction in fat grown-ups and teens, or overweight grown-ups with other weight-related clinical issues. Wegovy works by controlling craving and decreasing calorie consumption, prompting weight reduction and assisting with weight the executives.

Wegovy has a place with the class of medications called GLP-1 receptor agonists. GLP-1 receptor agonists are a produced rendition of GLP-1, a normally happening chemical in the body that demonstrations in a few regions in the mind to manage food consumption. At the point when Wegovy is directed, it actuates the GLP-1 receptors in the cerebrum. This brings down craving, lessening the calories consumed, prompting weight reduction.

his medication ought to be utilized along with a diminished calorie feast plan and expanded actual work to assist with weighting the executives.

Wegovy is given as an infusion under the skin (subcutaneous infusion) one time per week.

What is Wegovy utilized for?

Wegovy is a FDA-supported enemy of corpulence medication to be utilized by individuals 12 years and more established for ongoing weight the board when utilized along with a diminished calorie diet and expanded actual work.

Wegovy is shown for use in:

Grown-ups:

Stout (BMI of 30 kg/m2 or more prominent)

Overweight (BMI of 27 kg/m2 or more prominent) and have clinical issues (e.g. high pulse, type 2 diabetes, or elevated cholesterol) because of your weight.

Pediatric (12 years and more established):

Hefty (beginning BMI 95th percentile or more noteworthy for age and sex)

Wegovy contains semaglutide which is similar dynamic fixing in Ozempic and Rybelsus, subsequently these items ought not be utilized together. Ozempic (subcutaneous week after week infusion) and Rybelsus (once-a-day tablet) are utilized lower glucose levels for type two diabetic patients. Ozempic is additionally used to bring down the gamble of major cardiovascular occasions for some sort 2 diabetic patients.

Alerts

Call your primary care physician on the double on the off chance that you have indications of a thyroid growth, for example, expanding or an irregularity in your neck, inconvenience gulping, a rough voice, or windedness. In examinations with rodents, Wegovy and meds that work like Wegovy caused thyroid growths, including thyroid disease. It isn't known whether this medication will cause thyroid growths or a kind of thyroid disease called medullary thyroid carcinoma (MTC) in individuals.

You shouldn't utilize this medication on the off chance that you have growths in your organs called various endocrine neoplasia type 2 (MEN 2), or an individual or family background of medullary thyroid disease (MTC).

Prior to taking this medication

You shouldn't utilize Wegovy assuming you are:

susceptible to it or any of the fixings. See the finish of this page for a total rundown of fixings. Side effects of a serious hypersensitive response incorporate expanding of your face, lips, tongue, or throat, issues breathing or gulping, extreme rash or tingling, feeling woozy or unsteady, and an exceptionally quick heartbeat.

various endocrine neoplasia type 2 (growths in your organs); or

an individual or family background of medullary thyroid carcinoma (a sort of thyroid malignant growth).

Let your PCP know if you have at any point had:

a stomach or gastrointestinal issue;

pancreatitis;

kidney illness;

eye issues brought about by diabetes (diabetic retinopathy);

have or have had misery or self-destructive contemplations, or other emotional well-being issues.

In creature studies, semaglutide caused thyroid growths or thyroid disease. It isn't known whether these impacts would happen in individuals. Get some information about your gamble.

Pregnancy

You ought to quit utilizing this medication no less than two months before you intend to get pregnant. This medication might hurt your child. Ask your PCP for a more secure medication to use during this time. Controlling diabetes is vital during pregnancy, as is putting on the perfect proportion of weight. Regardless of whether you are overweight, getting thinner during pregnancy could hurt the unborn child.

There is a pregnancy openness library for ladies who use Wegovy during pregnancy. The justification behind this vault is to gather data about the strength of you and your child. Converse with your primary care physician about how you can participate in this vault, or you might contact Novo Nordisk at 1-800-727-6500.

Breastfeeding

Let your medical care proficient know if you are breastfeeding or wanting to breastfeed. It is obscure in the event that this medication passes into your bosom milk. You ought to consult with your medical services supplier about the most ideal way to take care of your child while utilizing this medication.

How could I utilize Wegovy?

Peruse the Guidelines for Utilize that is with your remedy and utilize this medication precisely as your medical care supplier tells you to. Your medical care supplier ought to prepare you on the most proficient method to utilize this medication before you begin utilizing it.

Wegovy is infused under the skin (subcutaneously) of your stomach (mid-region), thigh, or upper arm, utilizing a pen gadget. You shouldn't infuse this medication into a muscle (intramuscularly) or vein (intravenously).

This medication ought to be utilized one time every week, around the same time every week, whenever of the day.

You can take Wegovy regardless of food.

Set up an infusion just when you are prepared to give it. Call your drug specialist in the event that the medication looks overcast, has changed colors, or has particles in it.

In the event that you pick an alternate week by week infusion day, begin your new timetable after no less than two days have passed since the last infusion you gave.

Turn your infusion site with every infusion. You might infuse in a similar body region every week, except it is essential to utilize an alternate spot each time. Try not to infuse into a region where the skin is delicate, wounded, red, or hard. Try not to infuse into regions with scars or stretch imprints.

The Wegovy pen is for one-time utilize just, and the portion is as of now set on your pen.

The needle is covered by the needle cover and the needle won't be seen.

Eliminate the pen cap when you are prepared to infuse.

You shouldn't contact or push on the needle cover as you could get a needle stick injury.

To infuse, push the pen solidly against the skin and hold until the yellow bar has quit moving.

In the event that the yellow bar doesn't begin moving, you ought to press the pen all the more immovably against your skin.

You will hear two ticks during the infusion. Click 1 is the point at which the infusion has begun, and click two the infusion is as yet progressing.

Try not to eliminate the pen from your skin before the yellow bar in the pen window has quit moving. Assuming that you eliminate the needle prior, you may not get your full portion.

On the off chance that the yellow bar doesn't begin moving or quits during the infusion, contact your medical care supplier or Novo Nordisk at Wegovy.com or call Novo Nordisk Inc. at 1-833-934-6891.

The needle cover will lock when the pen is taken out from your skin. You can't stop the infusion and restart it later.

Put the utilized Wegovy pen in a FDA-cleared sharps removal compartment immediately after use. Try not to discard (discard) the pen in your family waste.

Individuals who are visually impaired or have vision issues shouldn't utilize the Wegovy pen without assistance from an individual prepared to utilize the pen.

Measurements

The portion begins low and heightens to limit gastrointestinal secondary effects.

Starting Portion Heightening Timetable for patients matured 12 years and more seasoned:

Weeks 1 through 4 (month one): 0.25 mg subcutaneously one time each week

Weeks 5 through 8 (month two): 0.5 mg subcutaneously one time each week

Weeks 9 through (year three): 1 mg subcutaneously one time each week

Weeks 13 through 16 (month four): 1.7 mg subcutaneously one time each week

Support Portion:

Week 17 and forward: 2.4 mg subcutaneously one time per week. See extra notes beneath about support dosing.

Upkeep Measurement Grown-up Patients. The upkeep measurement is 2.4 mg infused subcutaneously once week after week. In the event that the patient doesn't endure the upkeep 2.4 mg once-week after week dose, then, at that point, the dose can be briefly diminished to 1.7 mg one time each week, for a limit of about a month. Following a month, the portion ought to be expanded to the upkeep 2.4 mg once-week by week measurement. Stop this medication on the off chance that the patient can't endure the 2.4 mg measurement.

Pediatric Patients Matured 12 Years and More seasoned. The suggested support measurement of Wegovy is 2.4 mg infused subcutaneously once week by week. On the off chance that the patient doesn't endure the upkeep 2.4 mg once-week by week dose, the support measurement might be diminished to 1.7 mg once week after week. Suspend this medication on the off chance that the patient can't endure the 1.7 mg portion.

What occurs in the event that I miss a portion?

Utilize the medication at the earliest opportunity and afterward return to your standard timetable. Be that as it may, assuming that your next portion is expected in under two days (48 hours), avoid the missed portion and return to your customary timetable.

Call your primary care physician on the off chance that you miss multiple dosages in succession of Wegovy. You might have to restart the medication at a lower portion to keep away from stomach issues.

Try not to utilize two portions of semaglutide at one time.

What occurs assuming that I glut?

Look for crisis clinical consideration or call the Toxic Substance Help line at 1-800-222-1222.

Go too far may cause serious sickness, regurgitating, or low glucose.

What qualities is Wegovy accessible in?

Wegovy is accessible in five qualities:

Wegovy 0.25 mg (semaglutide) pen

Wegovy 0.5 mg (semaglutide) pen

Wegovy 1 mg (semaglutide) pen

Wegovy 1.7 mg (semaglutide) pen

Wegovy 2.4 mg(semaglutide) pen

General data

Try not to utilize various brands of semaglutide simultaneously.

Glucose can be impacted by pressure, ailment, medical procedure, work out, liquor use, or skipping feasts.

Low glucose (hypoglycemia) can cause you to feel exceptionally ravenous, tipsy, crabby, or insecure. To rapidly treat hypoglycemia, eat or drink hard sweets, wafers, raisins, natural product juice, or non-diet pop. Your PCP might recommend glucagon infusion if there should be an occurrence of extreme hypoglycemia.

Let your PCP know if you have successive side effects of high glucose (hyperglycemia), like expanded thirst or pee. Ask your PCP prior to changing your portion or prescription timetable.

Your therapy may likewise incorporate eating routine, work out, weight control, clinical trials, and extraordinary clinical consideration.

You might get dried out during drawn out ailment. Call your PCP in the event that you are debilitated with regurgitating or loose bowels or on the other hand assuming you eat or drink not exactly common.

What would it be a good idea for me to stay away from while utilizing Wegovy?

Never share an infusion pen, regardless of whether you changed the needle. Sharing this gadget can pass contamination or infection from one individual to another.

Wegovy incidental effects

Get crisis clinical assistance assuming you have indications of an unfavorably susceptible response: hives, tingling; unsteadiness, quick pulses, trouble breathing; expanding of your face, lips, tongue, or throat.

Semaglutide might cause serious secondary effects. Call your primary care physician without a moment's delay in the event that you have:

vision changes;

surprising mind-set changes, contemplations about harming yourself;

beating pulses or rippling in your chest;

a dazed inclination, similar to you could drop;

indications of a thyroid growth - enlarging or a bump in your neck, inconvenience gulping, a raspy voice, feeling winded;

side effects of pancreatitis- - serious agony in your upper stomach spreading to your back, sickness regardless of retching, quick pulse;

gallbladder issues - upper stomach torment, fever, mud shaded stools, jaundice (yellowing of the skin or eyes);

low glucose - migraine, hunger, shortcoming, perspiring, disarray, touchiness, unsteadiness, quick pulse, or feeling jumpy;

kidney issues - enlarging, peeing less, feeling drained or winded; or

stomach influenza side effects - stomach cramps, spewing, loss of hunger, the runs (might be watery or horrendous).

Normal results of semaglutide may include:

low glucose (in individuals with type 2 diabetes);

furious stomach, indigestion, burping, gas, bulging;

queasiness, spewing, stomach torment, loss of craving;

looseness of the bowels, blockage;

runny nose or sore throat;

stomach influenza side effects; o

cerebral pain, discombobulation, sluggishness.

What different medications will influence Wegovy?

Wegovy can slow your assimilation, and it might take more time for your body to ingest any medications you take by mouth.

Educate your primary care physician regarding all your different drugs, particularly insulin or other diabetes medication, for example, dulaglutide, exenatide, liraglutide, Byetta, Trulicity, Victoza, and others.

Different medications might influence Wegovy, including solution and over-the-counter prescriptions, nutrients, and natural items. Enlighten your primary care physician concerning any remaining drugs you use.

What are the fixings in Wegovy?

Dynamic Fixing: semaglutide

Dormant Fixings: disodium phosphate dehydrate, sodium chloride, and water for infusion

Producer

Wegovy is Fabricated by: Novo Nordisk A/S. Novo Allé. DK-2880 Bagsvaerd, Denmark.

Directions for Use

Before you utilize your Wegovy pen interestingly, converse with your medical services supplier or your parental figure about how to accurately get ready and infuse Wegovy.

Significant data

Peruse the Directions for Use before you begin utilizing Wegovy. This data doesn't supplant conversing with your medical care supplier about your ailment or therapy.

Your Wegovy pen is for one-time utilize as it were. The Wegovy pen is for subcutaneous (under the skin) utilize as it were.

The portion of Wegovy is as of now set on your pen.

The needle is covered by the needle cover and the needle won't be seen.

Try not to eliminate the pen cap until you are prepared to infuse.

Try not to contact or push on the needle cover. You could get a needle stick injury.

Your infusion will start when the needle cover is squeezed against your skin.

Try not to eliminate the pen from your skin before the yellow bar in the pen window has quit moving. Assuming the needle is taken out before, you may not get your full portion.

On the off chance that the yellow bar doesn't begin moving or quits during the infusion, contact your medical care supplier or Novo Nordisk at startWegovy.com or call Novo Nordisk Inc. at 1-833-934-6891.

The needle cover will lock when the pen is eliminated from your skin. You can't stop the infusion and restart it later.

Individuals who are visually impaired or have vision issues shouldn't utilize the Wegovy pen without assistance from an individual prepared to utilize the pen.

Step by step instructions to utilize your Wegovy pen

Try not to utilize your pen without getting preparing from your medical services supplier. Ensure that you or your guardian know how to give an infusion with the pen before you start your treatment.

Peruse and adhere to the guidelines with the goal that you utilize your pen accurately:

Stage 1. Plan for your infusion.

Supplies you should give your Wegovy infusion:

Wegovy pen

one liquor swab or cleanser and water

1 cloth cushion or cotton ball

1 sharps dispensable compartment

Clean up.

Check your Wegovy pen.

Try not to utilize your pen if:

The pen seems to have been utilized, or any piece of the pen seems broken, for instance, on the off chance that it has been dropped.

The Wegovy medication isn't clear and vapid through the pen window.

The lapse date (EXP) has passed.

Contact Novo Nordisk at 1-833-934-6891 in the event that your pen flops any of these checks.

Stage 2. Pick your infusion site.

Your medical services supplier can assist you with picking the infusion site that is best for you

You might infuse into your upper legs (front of the thighs) or lower stomach (keep 2 inches away from your paunch button).

Someone else may give the infusion in the upper arm.

Try not to infuse into a region where the skin is delicate, wounded, red, or hard. Try not to infuse into regions with scars or stretch imprints.

You might infuse in a similar body region every week, except ensure it isn't in a similar spot each time.

Clean the infusion site with a liquor swab or cleanser and water. Try not to contact the infusion site subsequent to cleaning.

Stage 3. Eliminate pen cap.

Pull the pen cap straight off your pen.

Stage 4. Infuse Wegovy.

Push the pen immovably against your skin until the yellow bar has quit moving.

On the off chance that the yellow bar doesn't begin moving, press the pen all the more solidly against your skin.

You will hear two ticks during the infusion.

Click 1: the infusion has begun.

Click 2: the infusion is continuous.

Stage 5. Discard (discard) pen.

Imagine a scenario in which blood shows up after infusion.

On the off chance that blood shows up at the infusion site, press the site gently with a dressing cushion or cotton ball.

How would I discard (discard) Wegovy pens?

Put the utilized Wegovy pen in a FDA-cleared sharps removal compartment immediately after use. Try not to discard (discard) the pen in your family junk.

In the event that you don't have a FDA-cleared sharps removal holder, you might utilize a family compartment that is:

made of a substantial plastic,

ready to be shut with a tight-fitting, cut safe top, without sharps having the option to emerge,

upstanding and stable during use,

release safe, and

appropriately named to caution of risky waste inside the holder.

At the point when your sharps removal compartment is practically full, you should adhere to your local area rules for the correct method for discarding your sharps removal holder.

Try not to reuse the pen.

Try not to reuse the pen or sharps removal holder or toss them into family garbage.

Significant: Keep your Wegovy pen, sharps removal compartment, and all drugs out of the compass of youngsters.

would I really focus on my pen?

Safeguard your pen:

Try not to drop your pen or thump it against hard surfaces.

Try not to open your pen to any fluids.

Assuming you imagine that your pen might be harmed, don't attempt to fix it. Utilize another one.

Keep the pen cap on until you are prepared to infuse. Your pen will as of now not be sterile in the event that you store an unused pen without the cap, on the off chance that you pull the pen cap off and put it on once more, or on the other hand assuming the pen cap is absent. This could prompt a disease.

General data about the protected and successful utilization of Wegovy.

Drugs are some of the time endorsed for purposes other than those recorded in a Prescription Aide. Try not to involve this medication for a condition for which it was not endorsed. Try not to give it to others, regardless of whether they have the very side effects that you have. It might hurt them. You can ask your drug specialist or medical services supplier for data that is composed for wellbeing experts.

Semaglutide (Wegovy, Ozempic, Rybelsus) is a medication utilized for weight reduction in unambiguous patients, and to bring down glucose levels and lessen the gamble of major cardiovascular occasions, for example, coronary episode or stroke in type two diabetes patients. Semaglutide is a GLP-1 agonist and works by expanding insulin discharge, bringing down how much glucagon delivered, postponing gastric exhausting and diminishing craving.

What is the distinction between Wegovy, Ozempic and Rybelus?

The various brands of semaglutide have various purposes and various structures:

Wegovy (subcutaneous infusion) is utilized for weight the executives for a particular gathering of patients and is given as a subcutaneous infusion week after week.

Ozempic (subcutaneous infusion) is utilized lower glucose levels for type two diabetic patients, alongside diet and exercise. It is additionally utilized for diabetic patients who as of now have cardiovascular sickness, to assist with bringing down the gamble of major cardiovascular occasions, for example, coronary failure or stroke. Ozempic is given as a subcutaneous infusion week by week.

Rybelsus (tablet) is utilized to bring down glucose levels for type two diabetic patients alongside diet and exercise, and is taken as a tablet one time per day.

Prior to taking this medication

You shouldn't utilize semaglutide assuming you are hypersensitive to it, or on the other hand in the event that you have:

numerous endocrine neoplasia type 2 (growths in your organs);

an individual or family background of medullary thyroid carcinoma (a sort of thyroid disease); or

diabetic ketoacidosis (call your PCP for treatment).

Let your PCP know if you have at any point had:

a stomach or digestive issue;

pancreatitis;

kidney infection; or

eye issues brought about by diabetes (retinopathy).

In creature studies, semaglutide caused thyroid growths or thyroid disease. It isn't known whether these impacts would happen in individuals. Get some information about your gamble.

People ought to quit utilizing semaglutide something like 2 months before you intend to get pregnant. Ask your PCP for a more secure medication to use during this time. Controlling diabetes is vital during pregnancy, as is putting on the perfect proportion of weight. Regardless of whether you are overweight, shedding pounds during pregnancy could hurt the unborn child.

Inquire as to whether it is protected to breastfeed while utilizing this Ozempic or Wegovy.

You shouldn't breastfeed while utilizing Rybelsus.

Semaglutide isn't endorsed for use by anybody more youthful than 18 years of age.

How does semaglutide work?

Semaglutide attempts to bring down high glucose by expanding how much insulin that is delivered, bringing down how much glucagon delivered and by deferring gastric purging. Semaglutide likewise controls hunger thus assists you with decreasing how much food that you need to eat. Semaglutide is a glucagon-like peptide-1 (GLP-1) agonist

How might I take semaglutide?

Wegovy and Ozempic are given as a subcutaneous infusion one time per week.

Rybelsus is a tablet that you require once a day toward the beginning of the day, 30 minutes prior to eating, drinking or taking some other prescriptions. You might eat, drink or take oral medication 30 minutes subsequent to taking Rybelsus

Dosing data:

Ozempic portion

Ozempic infusion 0.25 mg or 0.5 mg portion pen.

Pen can convey 0.25 mg or 0.5 mg dosages.

2mg/1.5mL (1.34mg/mL)

Each 1.5 ml pen contains 8 dosages of 0.25mg or 4 portions of 0.5mg.

Ozempic infusion 1 mg portion pen.

Pen conveys a 1mg portion.

4mg/3mL (1.34mg/mL)

Each 3ml pen contains 4 portions.

Ozempic infusion 2mg portion pen.

Pen conveys a 2mg portion.

8mg/3mL (2.68 mg/mL)

Each 3ml pen contains 4 dosages.

General semaglutide dosing data

Ozempic and Wegovy are infused under the skin, normally once each week whenever of the day, regardless of food. Utilize an infusion around the same time every week.

Peruse and adhere to all guidelines you have been given. Inquire as to whether you want assistance.

Set up an infusion just when you are prepared to give it. Call your drug specialist assuming the medication looks shady, has changed colors, or has particles in it.

Your medical care supplier will show you where to infuse semaglutide. Try not to infuse into similar spot twice in succession.

In the event that you pick an alternate week after week infusion day, begin your new timetable after something like 2 days have passed since the last infusion you gave.

Try not to utilize various brands of semaglutide simultaneously.

Glucose can be impacted by pressure, ailment, medical procedure, work out, liquor use, or skipping feasts.

Low glucose (hypoglycemia) can cause you to feel exceptionally eager, tipsy, peevish, or unsteady. To rapidly treat hypoglycemia, eat or drink hard sweets, saltines, raisins, natural product juice, or non-diet pop. Your PCP might endorse glucagon infusion if there should be an occurrence of serious hypoglycemia.

Let your PCP know if you have incessant side effects of high glucose (hyperglycemia) like expanded thirst or pee. Ask your primary care physician prior to changing your portion or medicine plan.

Your therapy may likewise incorporate eating regimen, work out, weight control, clinical trials, and unique clinical consideration.

You might get dried out during delayed sickness. Call your primary care physician assuming that you are debilitated with spewing or the runs, or on the other hand on the off chance that you eat or drink not exactly regular.

Store Rybelsus in the first bundle at room temperature, away from dampness and intensity.

Store unopened Ozempic or Wegovy infusion pens in the first container in a cooler, shielded from light. Try not to use past the termination date. Discard an infusion pen that has been frozen.

If necessary, you might store an unopened Wegovy pen at cool room temperature for as long as 28 days. Try not to eliminate the cap until you are prepared to utilize the infusion pen. The pen contains a solitary portion. Discard the pen after one use, regardless of whether there is still medication left inside.

The Ozempic infusion pen contains more than one portion. After your most memorable use, store the pen with the needle eliminated in a fridge or at room temperature. Shield from intensity and light. Keep the cap on when not being used. Discard the pen 56 days after the primary use, or on the other hand if under 0.25 mg is displayed on the portion counter.

Try not to reuse a needle. Place it in a cut resistant "sharps" compartment and discard it keeping state or nearby regulations. Keep out of the compass of youngsters and pets.

What occurs in the event that I miss a portion?

For Rybelsus: Avoid the missed portion and utilize your next portion at the customary time.

For Ozempic: Utilize the medication straightaway and afterward return to your customary timetable. Assuming you are over 5 days late for the infusion, avoid the missed portion and return to your ordinary timetable.

For Wegovy: Utilize the medication in a hurry and afterward return to your ordinary timetable. In the event that your next portion is expected in under 2 days (48 hours), avoid the missed portion and return to your normal timetable.

Try not to utilize two portions of semaglutide at one time.

Call your primary care physician in the event that you miss multiple dosages in succession of Wegovy. You might have to restart the medication at a lower portion to stay away from stomach issues.

What occurs assuming that I glut?

Look for crisis clinical consideration or call the Toxic Substance Help line at 1-800-222-1222.

Go too far may cause serious queasiness, heaving, or low glucose.

What would it be a good idea for me to keep away from while utilizing semaglutide?

Never share an infusion pen, regardless of whether you changed the needle. Sharing an infusion can pass contamination or sickness from one individual to another.

Semaglutide aftereffects

Get crisis clinical assistance in the event that you have indications of a hypersensitive response: hives, tingling; tipsiness, quick pulses; troublesome breathing; enlarging of your face, lips, tongue, or throat.

Serious symptoms of semaglutide may include:

call your PCP immediately in the event that you have:

vision changes;

uncommon mind-set changes, considerations about harming yourself;

beating pulses or shuddering in your chest;

a dazed inclination, similar to you could drop;

indications of a thyroid growth - enlarging or an irregularity in your neck, inconvenience gulping, a raspy voice, feeling winded;

side effects of pancreatitis- - serious agony in your upper stomach spreading to your back, queasiness regardless of spewing, quick pulse;

gallbladder issues - upper stomach torment, fever, dirt shaded stools, jaundice (yellowing of the skin or eyes);

low glucose - cerebral pain, hunger, shortcoming, perspiring, disarray, crabbiness, discombobulation, quick pulse, or feeling nervous;

kidney issues - expanding, peeing less, feeling drained or winded; or

stomach influenza side effects - stomach cramps, heaving, loss of craving, loose bowels (might be watery or ridiculous).

Normal symptoms of semaglutide may include:

low glucose (in individuals with type 2 diabetes);

furious stomach, acid reflux, burping, gas, bulging;

sickness, regurgitating, stomach torment, loss of craving;

the runs, blockage;

stomach influenza side effects; o

migraine, discombobulation, sluggishness.

What different medications will influence semaglutide?

Semaglutide can slow your assimilation, and it might take more time for your body to retain any drugs you take by mouth.

Educate your primary care physician concerning all your different prescriptions, particularly insulin or other diabetes medication, for example, dulaglutide, exenatide, liraglutide, Byetta, Trulicity, Victoza, and others.

Different medications might influence semaglutide, including remedy and over-the-counter prescriptions, nutrients, and natural items. Inform your PCP regarding any remaining drugs you use.

Pregnancy and breastfeeding

Pregnancy: People ought to quit utilizing semaglutide no less than 2 months before you intend to get pregnant. Ask your primary care physician for a more secure medication to use during this time. Controlling diabetes is vital during pregnancy, as is putting on the perfect proportion of weight. Regardless of whether you are overweight, getting more fit during pregnancy could hurt the unborn child.

Breastfeeding: Inquire as to whether it is protected to breastfeed while utilizing this Ozempic or Wegovy.

You shouldn't breastfeed while utilizing Rybelsus.

Capacity

Ozempic

Preceding first use, Ozempic ought to be put away in a fridge between 36ºF to 46ºF (2ºC to 8ºC). Try not to store in the cooler or straightforwardly adjoining the fridge cooling component. Try not to freeze Ozempic and don't utilize Ozempic assuming that it has been frozen.

After first utilization of the Ozempic pen, the pen can be put away for 56 days at controlled room temperature (59°F to 86°F; 15°C to 30°C) or in a fridge (36°F to 46°F; 2°C to 8°C). Try not to freeze.

Keep the pen cap on when not being used. Ozempic ought to be safeguarded from unreasonable intensity and daylight.

Continuously eliminate and securely dispose of the needle after every infusion and store the Ozempic pen without an infusion needle appended. Continuously utilize another needle for every infusion.

Wegovy

Store the single-portion pen in the fridge from 2°C to 8°C (36°F to 46°F). If necessary, preceding cap evacuation, the pen can be kept from 8°C to 30°C (46°F to 86°F) for as long as 28 days. Try not to freeze. Shield Wegovy from light. Wegovy should be kept in the first container until season of organization. Dispose of the Wegovy pen after use.

Saxenda (liraglutide) is utilized for weight reduction and to assist with keeping weight off whenever weight has been lost, it is utilized for corpulent grown-ups or overweight grown-ups who additionally have weight-related clinical issues. Saxenda can be utilized in kids matured 12 to 17 years who with corpulence and who have a bodyweight over 132 pounds (60 kg). Saxenda is utilized along with a sound eating regimen and exercise.

Saxenda is an infusion allowed once a day under the skin (subcutaneous) from a multi-portion infusion pen.

Saxenda contains a similar dynamic fixing (liraglutide) as Victoza. The distinction among Saxenda and Victoza is they are various qualities and they are FDA supported for various circumstances.

Saxenda isn't for treating type 1 or type 2 diabetes. It isn't known whether Saxenda is protected and successful in kids under 12 years old. It isn't known whether Saxenda is protected and compelling in youngsters matured 12 to 17 years with type 2 diabetes.

How does Saxenda function?

Saxenda attempts to assist with weighting misfortune by bringing down craving, easing back gastric discharging which encourages you for longer and accordingly you decline your calorie consumption. Saxenda is like a chemical that happens normally in the body and assists control with blooding sugar, insulin levels, and processing. Saxenda has a place with a class of medications called glucagon-like peptide-1 (GLP-1) agonists.

What is Saxenda utilized for?

Saxenda is FDA supported for weight reduction and to assist with keeping weight off whenever you have shed pounds. It tends to be utilized for:

Grown-ups:

corpulent grown-ups (BMI 30 kg/m2 or more prominent)

overweight grown-ups (BMI 27 kg/m2 or more prominent) who additionally have weight-related clinical issues e.g., hypertension, type 2 diabetes mellitus, or dyslipidemia.

Pediatric patients matured 12 years and more seasoned:

body weight over 60 kg and

their underlying BMI relating to 30 kg/m2 or more noteworthy for grown-ups (fat) by global shorts (Cole Standards)

Admonitions

The Victoza brand of liraglutide is utilized along with diet and exercise to treat type 2 diabetes. Try not to utilize Saxenda and Victoza together.

You shouldn't utilize Saxenda in the event that you have various endocrine neoplasia type 2 (growths in your organs), an individual or family background of medullary thyroid disease, insulin-subordinate diabetes, diabetic ketoacidosis, or are pregnant.

In creature studies, liraglutide caused thyroid growths or thyroid disease. It isn't known whether these impacts would happen in individuals utilizing standard dosages.

Call your primary care physician without a moment's delay in the event that you have indications of a thyroid cancer, for example, expanding or a bump in your neck, inconvenience gulping, a raspy voice, or windedness.

Prior to utilizing Saxenda

You shouldn't utilize Saxenda assuming you are sensitive to liraglutide, or on the other hand in the event that you have:

various endocrine neoplasia type 2 (cancers in your organs);

an individual or family background of medullary thyroid carcinoma (a kind of thyroid malignant growth); or diabetic ketoacidosis (call your primary care physician for treatment).

You shouldn't utilize Saxenda assuming you additionally use insulin or different drugs like liraglutide (albiglutide, dulaglutide, exenatide, Byetta, Bydureon, Tanzeum, Trulicity).

To ensure Saxenda is alright for you, let your PCP know if you have:

stomach issues causing slow processing;

kidney or liver illness;

high fatty substances (a kind of fat in the blood);

heart issues;

a background marked by issues with your pancreas or gallbladder; or

a background marked by misery or self-destructive contemplations.

In creature studies, liraglutide caused thyroid growths or thyroid disease. It isn't known whether these impacts would happen in individuals utilizing ordinary portions. Get some information about your gamble.

It isn't known whether Saxenda will hurt an unborn child. Let your PCP know if you are pregnant or want to become pregnant.

It isn't known whether liraglutide passes into bosom milk or on the other hand on the off chance that it could influence the nursing child. Let your PCP know if you are bosom taking care of.

Printed in Great Britain
by Amazon